The Dukan Diet: Lose Weight Quickly and Safely for Life with the Dukan Diet Plan

BENJAMIN TIDEAS

CONTENTS

INTRODUCTION

I want to thank you and congratulate you on purchasing the book, "The Dukan Diet: Lose Weight Quickly and Safely for Life with the Dukan Diet Plan".

This book contains proven steps and strategies on how to finally lose the weight you've wanted with the Dukan Diet. More importantly, is the focus on keeping that weight off for good. There are obviously many diet plans available to anyone wanting to shed those extra pounds. The questions that arise are: which diets are safe, which diets produce rapid results, and which diets will provide lasting results? Also, of course, which diet is right for my plan and my lifestyle? This book aims to answer those questions, give you specifics, arm you with resources and show you just how effectively the Dukan diet can work for you.

Thanks again for buying this book, I hope you enjoy it! Now, let's get to it!

UNDERSTANDING THE DUKAN DIET

The Dukan diet is unlike other diets that have come and gone. Although it bears some similarities with other high-protein, low-carbohydrate diets, this particular diet is unique, simply because it is not one-size-fits-all. Each person needs to set a target weight that is based on one's "true weight". One's "true weight" is where that person is at his or her healthiest. Some people may be disappointed that their "true age" doesn't correspond with their ideal weight. In calculating a person's "true weight", this diet method takes the differences in people's bodies into consideration.

Some of the factors that affect one's "true weight" are the person's age, sex, body type, and previous diets he or she has tried in the past. The Dukan diet is designed to help people lose weight quickly without having to count calories or limit the amount of food they eat in a day. The idea of losing weight without having to starve oneself is one of the diet's main selling points; however, this is just the tip of the iceberg. Aside from astounding weight loss results, the Dukan diet also promises to help in maintaining one's ideal weight for as long as that person follows the diet.

Another thing that makes the Dukan diet different is the phases that people on this diet need to go through. It's not a one-time-big-time weight loss plan that other diets promise. If a person follows the diet until the very last phase, the risk of regaining all the pounds that have been lost is significantly reduced, if not eliminated. The diet is divided into 4 phases – the attack phase, the cruise phase, the consolidation phase, and lastly, the stabilization phase. The first two phases deal with losing weight, while the last two are meant to help the body adjust to the diet and make a lifestyle change in order to maintain a healthy weight.

The road to a slimmer, healthier body isn't an easy one. Despite having no limits in the number of calories that can be consumed in a day, the Dukan diet has a lot of rules and restrictions, especially in the early phases. This does mellow down towards the last phase of the diet when the target weight has been met, and maintenance is the only goal. The Dukan diet also prescribes physical activity and exercise to go with the diet. The exercise aspect of this weight loss plan is also personalized and could include a 20-minute walk or something more strenuous depending on the person's fitness level.

The Dukan diet was developed by Pierre Dukan, a French physician who has been helping people lose weight for over 25 years now. He came up with this diet program after he was able to help one of his patients lose 10 lbs in five days without cutting meat out of his diet. From there, he began to develop the Dukan diet phase by phase and has since written 19 books on the subject of weight loss.

For most of his career, Dr. Dukan was a household name in France when it came to weight loss. He has helped countless people in his home country lose weight and keep the weight off. It was only a matter of time before he shared his methods to the rest of the world. His most popular book to date is The Dukan Diet, which was published in 2000. In this book, he divulges the secrets to successful weight loss and weight maintenance. This book has also brought the diet method he has painstakingly developed over the years to the international stage.

Like other diets that promote high protein and low carbohydrate intake, the Dukan diet has faced some resistance from certain nutrition experts who insist that limiting calorie intake is still the best method for losing weight. This is despite the fact that the problem concerning obesity has been increasing continuously and exponentially over the years. In spite of all the criticism, Pierre Dukan stands by his process and aims to change the way the world tackles the problem of obesity.

WHAT TO EXPECT WITH THE DUKAN DIET

There are many words one can use to describe the Dukan diet, but "easy" isn't one of them. It takes a lot of discipline to stay on track when trying out any diet, and the Dukan diet is no exception to this rule. In fact, many online diet reviews describe this diet as a "stricter" version of some of the most popular low-carb, high-protein diets. For those who are interested in going on the Dukan diet, here are some things one should expect:

Personalized diet plans – The Dukan diet is not a one-size-fits-all diet that one can just plunge into whenever he or she feels like it. Before starting the diet, one should first calculate his or her "true weight", which takes a lot of different factors into account. Once a person's "true weight" is established, it would be easier to determine one's weight loss target and how long to stay in each phase.

No calorie-counters – The most appealing aspect of the Dukan diet is the fact that it allows dieters to eat as much as they want in a day provided that they only eat the foods that are allowed for each phase. This means that a person on this diet won't have to starve his or herself even during the attack phase which is where most of the weight loss happens.

Protein, protein, and more protein – The core of the Dukan diet is protein. There are around 68 different types of protein-rich food items which are the only ones allowed during the attack phase. By the time the dieter reaches the cruise phase, low-carb vegetables are slowly introduced into the diet plan.

Fat is a no-no – Unlike other low-carb diets, the amount of fat intake is very limited with the Dukan diet. Dairy products are allowed as long as they are fat-free. Olive oil is also allowed but only in very limited quantities.

More water, please – A person on the Dukan diet is expected to drink 1.5 liters of water a day at the very least. Eating all that protein may cause a spike in uric acid production and so more water is needed to keep one's vital organs running properly. Tea and coffee are acceptable, and in some cases, so is diet soda. Alcoholic beverages are not allowed while one is in the first three stages of the Dukan diet. Aside from alcohol, fruit juices and regular soda are also not allowed.

It will get easier – The Dukan diet is very strict in terms of what a person is allowed to eat in the first three stages; however, each stage is more lenient than the previous stage. By the time a dieter reaches the last phase – the stabilization phase – dieters can relax a bit and have the freedom to eat whatever they want – except on Pure Protein Thursdays when dieters go back to the attack phase. The freedom to eat whatever they want (including foods that are high in fat or carbohydrates) comes with a great deal of responsibility. Going back to old eating habits will only negate all the progress made. The best thing to do during this phase is to maintain sensible eating habits in order to stay within one's "true weight".

Exercise – Many people are surprised to hear that exercise is a part of the Dukan diet plan, but it makes sense. Just as gym instructors often advise their clients on what they should eat and what they should avoid, the Dukan diet also promotes exercise as part of the diet regimen. The reason for this is that limiting the food one consumes isn't enough for optimum weight loss. Lack of physical activity also makes it hard for a dieter to maintain their weight once they reach their weight loss goals. The Dukan diet recommends an average of 20 minutes of physical activity daily (more during the cruise phase to prevent gaining back the weight lost in the attack phase). Aside from cardiovascular exercises, people on the Dukan diet can also change it up a bit and add some strengthening and muscle toning exercises for a stronger, more proportioned body.

DUKAN DIET PHASES

The problem with most diets is that once a person reaches his or her target weight and goes off the diet, they tend to gain it all back and then some. The Dukan diet addresses this concern by dividing the entire process into 4 phases. Each phase serves its own purpose in helping dieters lose weight and keep the pounds off for life. The 4 phases are:

1) The Attack Phase – The goal of this first phase is to jumpstart one's weight loss. This is the shortest phase, and yet it is the most difficult, especially for people who are used to eating foods that are high in sugar, fat, and carbohydrates. During the attack phase, dieters are only allowed to eat lean meats and other foods that are rich in protein. There are 68 different types of food that are allowed during this phase. The duration of the attack phase varies from 2-7 days depending on what the dieter's target weight is.

Weight Loss Expectations during the Attack Phase: It is in the attack phase that dieters lose a lot of weight in a short period. The idea is to kick start one's metabolism and shed anywhere from 4-6 pounds a day. This makes it easier for the body to continue losing weight. The staggering results also help encourage people to stay on the diet and see it through until the end.

2) The Cruise Phase – It is in this phase that a dieter works to reach his or her true weight. After the rapid weight loss that occurs in the attack phase, this next phase slows things down a little. Weight loss is still expected, but not as drastic as in the initial stage of the diet. By this time, a dieter can start adding any of the 32 prescribed vegetables to their diet. Dieters are encouraged to alternate protein and vegetable days with pure protein days to get the best effect. The cruise phase lasts for as long as the dieter has not achieved his true weight.

Weight Loss Expectations during the Cruise Phase: Weight loss slows down considerably during the cruise phase of the Dukan diet. The expected weight loss would be one pound every three to seven days depending on conditions that are specific to each person who is on this diet.

3) The Consolidation Phase – This is the part of the Dukan diet that is missing in other similar diet plans. At this stage, a dieter's body is susceptible to regaining all the weight he or she has lost in the first two phases. During this phase, foods that were previously banned in the attack and cruise phases are slowly reintroduced. Dieters are also allowed to have two "celebratory meals" each week. Being able to eat foods that were previously disallowed doesn't mean that the diet ends here. Every Thursday is still considered a PP day or Pure Protein day where one should only eat foods that are allowed during the attack phase. This phase follows a rigid schedule. Every pound lost during the cruise phase is equivalent to 5 days on the consolidation phase. For example, if a dieter loses 10 lbs in the cruise phase, he or she must stay on the consolidation phase for 50 days.

Weight Loss Expectations during the Consolidation Phase: By the time the dieter gets to the consolidation phase, he or she has already achieved their target weight. The goal of this phase is not to lose any more weight, but to make sure it doesn't come back. Gaining a pound or two in the beginning is not a cause for worry. It should stabilize as the dieter continues on in this phase.

4) The Stabilization Phase – When entering this phase, think of it as a graduation of sorts. All the excess weight has been eliminated, and it has been kept off for several weeks or months after reaching one's target weight. This is where the real challenge begins. The first 3 phases of the Dukan diet have already altered a dieter's eating habits. The hope is that although the dieters are free to eat whatever they want, they will still choose to maintain healthy eating habits. Dieters in this phase are still required to maintain the Pure Protein Thursday habit and eat 3 Tbsp of oat bran daily. 20 minutes of exercise per day is also a requirement. If a dieter maintains this, chances are, he or she won't have problems with weight ever again.

Weight Loss Expectations during the Stabilization Phase: This is a long term phase that requires dedication. If a dieter doesn't go off the reservation when in this phase, then weight gain won't be a problem. On the other hand, if the dieter forgets to eat responsibly and completely ditches the Pure Protein Thursday, weight gain is definitely possible.

FOOD LIST AND DIET PLANS

The Dukan diet plan is quite simple. Only certain foods are allowed in each phase of the diet. As the dieter goes through each phase and eventually reaches his or her "true weight", the diet plan gets less and less restrictive. Slowly, other foods are introduced starting with vegetables that are on the "allowed list" for the cruise phase and other previously banned food items can be introduced into the diet when the dieter reaches the consolidation phase. This goes on until the final phase where the dieter is free to eat anything he or she wants. There is a catch, however. Once the dieter is on the stabilization phase of the Dukan diet, he or she must reserve one day (Thursday) where he or she will follow an attack phase meal plan of only pure proteins. The dieter must also eat 3 tablespoons of oat bran a day and must also maintain a 20-minute exercise regimen daily.

The Dukan Diet Food List:

While developing this revolutionary diet plan, Dr. Dukan was able to identify 68 Pure Protein foods and 32 vegetables that not only help with weight loss, but also add nutritional value to the diet. All these foods are low in fat and carbohydrates and are high in protein, as well.

The Dukan diet can be very restrictive, especially during the first two phases. Beginners may find it hard to eliminate carbohydrates at first, especially if they are staples in one's diet, but the 68 proteins and 32 vegetables are more than enough to make up for it in terms of variety and taste.

The 68 pure proteins are the heart of the first phase of the Dukan diet People can choose to have any of the following food during the attack phase:

- Lean meats like sirloin, beef tenderloin, pork tenderloin, veal chops, venison, pork loin roast and other low-fat cuts of meat.
- Poultry food items like chicken, turkey, quail, wild duck and other poultry food products (chicken/turkey hotdogs and sausages. turkey ham, etc…). This category also includes chicken, quail and duck eggs.
- Certain types of fish like sardines, mackerel, salmon, halibut, red snapper, tilapia, swordfish, tuna, and trout, among others.
- Other seafood including crabs, mussels, octopus, crayfish, crawfish, shrimp, squid, oysters, and scallops.
- Dairy products like milk, cottage cheese, cream cheese, sour cream, ricotta cheese, and Greek yogurt are allowed provided that they are of the fat-free variety.
- Vegetable proteins like food products made out of soy (tofu, veggie burgers, etc…).

After the attack phase, people who are on the Dukan diet can now re-introduce vegetables into their diet. The 32 types of vegetables allowed during the cruise phase are:

Broccoli
Cauliflower
Artichoke
Bean Sprouts
Asparagus
Brussels' Sprouts
Beets
Celery
Carrot
Eggplant
Cucumber
Onions
Radicchio
Fennel
Endive
Green Beans
Palm Hearts
Leeks
Arugula
Lettuce
Kale
Shallots
Okra
Watercress
Peppers
Spinach
Turnip
Zucchini
Radishes
Pumpkin
Squash
Spaghetti Squash

Aside from these core foods, other food items allowed in the Dukan diet include sugar-free gelatin, goji berries, olive oil and Shirataki noodles which have zero carbohydrates and can replace pasta. Natural sweeteners like Organic Stevia can be used to sweeten drinks like coffee and tea.

People on the Dukan diet are encouraged to take multivitamins in order to make up for nutrients lost by limiting the types of food one can eat. Drinking lots of water is also advised to prevent the buildup of uric acid in the body as a result of eating only proteins.

CHECKING YOUR PROGRESS

Progress – that's the magic word that all dieters want to hear. No matter what diet they're on, all the hard work and sacrifice becomes worth it when they start seeing results. With the Dukan diet, progress can be seen almost immediately. Here are some tips for tracking one's weight loss progress.

The scale is your friend, not an enemy – All a person needs to check his or her progress while on the Dukan diet is a weighing scale. Before going on a diet, standing on a scale, can be frightening, but knowing one's starting weight is important when tracking one's progress. Seeing the numbers whenever one steps on the scale is a clear indication that the diet is indeed working. Of course, weighing one's self every day is not advisable, except during the attack phase, where pounds are expected to drop on a daily basis.

When weighing one's self daily, it is advisable to step on the scale around the same time every day. This is done in order to make sure that things like water retention don't factor into the numbers the scale displays. For more accurate results, a weekly weigh-in would tell a dieter just how much progress he or she has made after weeks or months of dieting. Creating a weight loss chart to keep track of one's progress is also a good idea.

Take "selfies" – Numbers don't lie, but mirrors often do. Even after losing 10 lbs, people can feel like nothing has changed when they look at themselves in the mirror. One way to visually track one's weight loss progress is through taking "selfies." A selfie is a picture of a person taken by him or herself. Face the mirror and begin taking "before" photos of your reflection. Make sure to snap a few shots at the end of every week until the target weight is reached. Once you reach your "true weight", collect all the pictures and arrange them in order. It's often very stunning to see just how much of a difference losing those 5 to 10 lbs make in one's appearance.

Get a Dukan Diet Coach – People who are serious about losing weight through the Dukan diet can go the extra mile and sign up for an interactive personal coach on the Dukan diet website. A coaching subscription allows dieters to fill out a progress report which they will submit to their coach also via the website. The coach tracks the person's progress and provides personalized diet plans that would address any problems that would arise such as lack of physical activity, frustrations while on the diet, and weight loss issues, among others. Coaching also makes it easy for the dieter to determine whether he or she should stay in the phase they are in, or move on to the next phase.

HOW TO STAY MOTIVATED ON THE DUKAN DIET

When people go on a diet, they expect to see results – and fast. Results are what keep dieters motivated. The more they lose, the more likely they will stick to the diet. The first few days of a new diet are crucial, and if one loses a significant amount of weight at the beginning of a diet, the more motivated a person becomes to do what it takes in order to shed whatever is left of the excess weight. That's why the attack phase is designed the way it is. People on the attack phase of the Dukan diet usually lose anywhere between 4-6 lbs a day. If that's not motivation enough, then what is?

The succeeding phases tell a different story, however. The amount of weight loss that can be achieved during the cruise phase drops significantly as vegetables are re-introduced into the diet. It may take more time for the body to get rid of all the extra weight that was left behind after the attack phase, but the weight loss isn't over yet. This may be disappointing for some people who have gotten used to seeing their weight plummet whenever they step on the scale; however, being on the cruise phase means that the dieter is getting closer and closer to his or her "true weight." This decrease in the amount of weight loss shouldn't discourage a dieter. In fact, it should be considered a challenge to stick more closely to the diet plan. The phase where people usually jump ship is the consolidation phase. The added temptation of being allowed to eat certain foods that were once banned from the diet makes it difficult to stay on track. In addition, this phase is all about maintenance and weight loss won't be a factor anymore.

Motivation is a significant factor when it comes to how successful a diet plan can be. If one is not motivated, the tendency is to cheat or to quit the diet altogether. When this happens, all the hard work done in the past few days, weeks, or months goes down the drain. This is why it is important to keep things fresh. Here are some tips for staying motivated while on the Dukan diet:

- Create a progress chart – Charting one's progress serves as a reminder of how much more weight a dieter still needs to lose. It shows how much weight a person has lost in a particular period. When the scale seems to be saying otherwise, a progress chart serves as a reminder that progress is being made.

- Find support – When giving up seems to be the only way to end one's diet frustrations, a support system would surely come in handy. It could be a friend, a family member, or a loved one who supports the dieter's decision to shed the extra weight and live a healthy life. These people can provide words of encouragement or even act as the dieter's conscience every time he or she feels like falling off the wagon. It would also be better if friends and family members go on the Dukan diet, as well. This way, it won't be frustrating to watch people eat carbohydrate-rich foods while sticking to pure proteins

- A reward for progress – Achieving one's "true weight" is already a reward in itself, but what about those moments when a dieter achieves a short term weight loss target? Reaching weekly or monthly weight loss goals is a significant achievement and like most achievements in life, it deserves a reward. Unfortunately, many people think that a "reward" after losing 10 lbs would be to have that sinfully delicious slice of chocolate cake. That's not a reward; that's cheating. The reward in this case could be anything from a new pair of shoes, a relaxing day at the spa, or anything that would motivate a dieter to achieve his or her goals.

- Mix it up – Just because the Dukan diet allows only 100 types of food, it doesn't mean that a dieter's meal plan should revolve around just a few dishes. There are many Dukan recipes from which to choose. All it takes is a little imagination to have delicious Dukan-approved meals every single day.

Move, move, move – Exercise is not a suggestion in the Dukan diet; it's a requirement. Aside from burning calories, adding a 20-30 minute exercise regimen helps the body metabolize food faster. The extra pounds lost with the aid of exercise will be more than enough motivation to keep at it.

CONCLUSION

I want to personally Thank You again for purchasing this book!

I sincerely hope the information contained will help you to understand the benefits of the Dukan Diet. More importantly, I hope that you feel ready to finally lose those unwanted pounds using the resources we have discussed.

The next step is to put into practice the methods and employ the strategies we've discussed here to begin losing that weight for good!

Please enjoy the bonus recipe section to follow that we've compiled for your convenience.

Finally, if you enjoyed this book, please take the time to share your thoughts and post a positive review on Amazon. I would greatly appreciate your support!

Visit me online at: http://www.plaid-enterprises.com/benjamin-tideas

Thank you and good luck!

Benjamin Tideas

ATTACK PHASE RECIPES

CREAMY CHICKEN WITH TOASTED PARMESAN

Ingredients:
- 2 chicken breasts, cut into 1-1/2 inch cubes
- 6 oz plain Greek yogurt
- 1/2 tsp onion powder
- 1/2 tsp garlic salt
- 1 tsp Italian seasoning
- 4 tbs parmesan
- dash of black pepper & chili powder

Directions:
1. Preheat oven 375 F.
2. Mix chicken breast, Greek yogurt, garlic salt, onion powder, Italian seasoning, and 2 tbs parmesan in a bowl.
3. Pour mixture into an oven-safe dish and bake for 35 minutes.
4. While the chicken bakes, combine remaining parmesan, black pepper, and chili powder in a small bowl.
5. Lay parchment paper on a baking sheet and spoon the parmesan mix into 2 mounds onto the parchment paper.
6. Use the back of the spoon to flatten the mounds. Add the parmesan to the oven during the last 6-8 minutes of the chicken's baking time until the parmesan is golden brown.
7. Crumble the remaining parmesan on top.

CHICKEN FAJITA STRIPS

Ingredients:
- 1 lb chicken breast
- 1 packet chicken fajita seasoning
- 8 oz roasted red peppers (fresh or from the jar)
- 1/2 white onion, sliced
- 1/2 tbs minced garlic

Directions:
1. Slice chicken breasts into 1-inch strips and place in a bowl.
2. Spray the chicken with cooking spray for one second and add the fajita seasoning (leave 1-2 tablespoons of seasoning for the vegetables). Use your hands to rub the seasoning into the chicken.
3. Preheat a pan over medium heat or indoor grill at 350F with cooking spray.
4. Place the chicken strips on the cooking surface and cook for about 2 minutes on each side. Set the chicken to the side.
5. Preheat a pan over medium heat with cooking spray. Add garlic and saute until fragrant.
6. Add onions and 1/2 of the remaining seasoning and cook until they begin to soften. Stir in roasted red peppers and the rest of the seasoning and cook for 1 minute.

Add the chicken into the pan with the vegetables to combine and reheat the chicken. You can also use fresh bell peppers instead of the canned. Of course, you would have to cook fresh bell peppers for a bit longer. Omit the vegetables for attack phase or pure protein days.

SIRLOIN W/ PARMESAN CREAM SAUCE

Ingredients:
- 2 lbs top sirloin
- salt & pepper to taste
- 1/2 cup finely chopped onion
- 2 cloves garlic, minced
- 1/2 cup fat free cream cheese
- 1 cup low-fat Parmesan cheese
- 1 cup fat free half & half
- 1/8 teaspoon ground black pepper
- 1 tbs chopped fresh parsley

Directions:
1. Season steaks with salt, pepper, and any other desired steak seasoning.
2. Grill for 2-4 per side or 4-7 in a Foreman Grill depending on how well you like your steak.
3. Heat a medium pan with cooking spray on medium heat.
4. Add garlic and onions and saute for about 1 minute.
5. Add cream cheese, half & half, and parmesan cheese. Stir over heat until cheese is melted and smooth.
6. Add salt & pepper to taste and finish with parsley and remove from heat.

BUFFALO CHICKEN

Ingredients:
- 3 boneless, skinless chicken breasts (cut into 1 inch cubes or strips)
- 1/2 cup Frank's Red Hot Sauce
- 3/4 cup fat free chicken broth
- 1 tbs corn starch, dissolved in 1 tbs chicken broth

Directions:
1. Heat medium pot with cooking spray and brown chicken.
2. In a bowl, stir together chicken broth and hot sauce. Pour sauce into pot.
3. Allow chicken to simmer in sauce for 14 minutes.
4. Whisk in corn starch, bring to a boil, and remove from heat.

To make a **low-fat ranch sauce** for dipping, buy a packet of dry Hidden Valley Ranch mix. Prepare according to package directions with low-fat mayo and skim milk.

CHOCOLATE MOLTEN LAVA CAKE

Ingredients:
- 3 tbs unflavored protein powder
- 2 tsp cocoa powder
- 1 egg
- 2 tbs splenda brown sugar
- 1/4 tsp vanilla extract
- 1 tbs skim milk
- 2 tbs oat bran
- 1 tsp baking powder
- dash of salt
- 1-2 tbs sugar-free chocolate sauce

Directions:
1. Preheat oven 350 F.
2. Whisk all ingredients together and pour into a souffle cup.
3. Bake for 15-18 minutes. (the outside rim should be cooked while the center remains very moist)
4. Pour sugar-free chocolate sauce over cake and serve while hot.

CRUISE PHASE RECIPES

ROSEMARY CHICKEN & ROASTED VEGETABLES

Ingredients:
- 4 chicken breast halves
- 2 cups broccoli or bell peppers
- 1 zucchini, cut into cubes
- 1/2 medium onion, chopped
- 2 cloves garlic, minced
- mix together a few dashes of: salt, pepper, rosemary, garlic powder, and onion powder.

Directions:
1. Preheat oven 350 F.
2. Lightly sprinkle dry seasoning mix on both sides of chicken breasts.
3. Heat pan on medium-high heat with cooking spray.
4. Brown chicken breasts on both sides (do not cook through).
5. Meanwhile, place vegetables in a medium baking dish with dry seasoning mix and cooking spray and toss together.
6. Remove chicken from pan and place chicken on top of vegetables.
7. Bake for 35-45 minutes.

JALAPEÑO CHEESE CHICKEN

Ingredients:
- 4 chicken breast halves
- 3 tbs fat free cheddar/mozzarella cheese
- 3 oz fat free cream cheese
- 2 jalapeños, cleaned & minced
- salt & pepper

Directions:
1. Preheat oven 375 F.
2. Place plastic wrap over chicken breasts and flatten with a mallet.
3. Season chicken with salt & pepper on one side and flip over.
4. Mix together cheeses and minced jalapenos.
5. Spread jalapeno cheese mixture onto chicken breasts.
6. Roll chicken and hold with a toothpick.
7. Spray cooking spray on baking sheet, place chicken, and top with more spray.
8. Bake for 30 minutes.

SMOKED TURKEY JAMBALAYA

Ingredients:
- 14 oz lean smoked turkey sausage, sliced
- 3/4 cup chopped celery
- 3/4 cup chopped onion
- 3/4 cup chopped green bell peppers
- 2 tbs minced garlic
- 1 cup diced tomatoes
- 3 bay leaves
- 1 tsp hot sauce
- 1 tsp Worcestershire sauce
- 2-1/2 cups fat free chicken broth
- Combine a dash of each of the following spices: paprika, black pepper, chili powder, onion powder, garlic powder, oregano, & thyme.

Directions:
1. Heat a large sauce pan on medium heat with cooking spray and brown onions, celery, and bell peppers for 3 minutes.
2. Add tomatoes, garlic, bay leaves, Worcestershire sauce, and hot sauce.
3. Slowly add chicken broth.
4. Cover and cook for 20 minutes. Stir occasionally.
5. In a separate pan, spray with cooking spray and brown sausage. Set aside.
6. Remove cover and cook 15 minutes.
7. Mix in sausage and spice-mix and cook for an additional few minutes.

CORNED BEEF AND CABBAGE

Ingredients:
- 1.5 lb tri-tip roast (fat trimmed)
- 5 large wedges of cabbage
- 3 tbs kosher salt
- 1/2 large white onion quartered
- 1 tbs pickling spice
- 1/8 cup splenda brown sugar
- 1 tsp minced garlic
- 1 tsp black pepper

Directions:
Combine all ingredients in a crock pot and add water to barely cover the roast. Set the crock pot on low for 8 hours.

CINNAMON ROLL PUDDING

Ingredients:
- 3/4 tsp vanilla extract
- 1/2 cup fat free cream cheese
- 1/2 cup soft tofu
- 3 packets of splenda
- 1 tbs splenda brown sugar
- 1/2 tsp ground cinnamon

Directions:
1. Blend all ingredients together in a food processor or blender until smooth.
2. Refrigerate for a few hours for a thick consistency.

CONSOLIDATION PHASE RECIPES

LEMON GARLIC SHRIMP

Ingredients:
- 1 lb shrimp, deveined
- 1/4 lemon
- 3 cloves garlic, minced
- salt & pepper to taste

Directions:
1. In a pan, heat cooking spray on medium.
2. Add garlic and cook until fragrant.
3. Add shrimp and squeeze lemon over the shrimp.
4. Add salt and pepper to taste. Cook until shrimp is cooked through.
5. Optional: add red pepper flakes if you like it spicy.

CHICKEN WITH ROSEMARY CREAM SAUCE

Ingredients:
- 4 chicken breast halves
- 1/2 cup fat free chicken broth
- 1/2 cup chopped green onions
- 1 tsp fresh rosemary – minced
- 1/4 cup white wine
- 1/2 cup fat free half and half
- salt and pepper

Directions:
1. Heat pan over medium heat with cooking spray.
2. Season both sides of chicken breasts with salt and pepper.
3. Add chicken to pan and cook for 3 minutes per side.
4. Add green onions, wine, and rosemary and cook for 30 seconds.
5. Add chicken broth and cook for 2 minutes.
6. Stir in half and half and cook for 2 minutes.

Note: This is a thin, light cream sauce. If you prefer your sauce thicker, dissolve a tsp or two of cornstarch in hot water and add it to the sauce. Heat it to the simmer and take it off the stove to thicken.

SHREDDED CHICKEN LETTUCE WRAPS

Ingredients:
- 3 chicken breasts
- 16 oz chunky salsa
- 3-5 tbs fat free cream cheese
- Iceberg lettuce

Directions:
1. Combine chicken and salsa in a crock pot.
2. Cook on low for 8 hours.
3. Strain out half of the juices. Shred chicken using a fork.
4. Mix in 3-5 tbs of cream cheese depending on how thick you like the sauce.
5. Serve with iceberg lettuce leaves.

PESTO-RUBBED TRI-TIP

Ingredients:
- 3 lbs tri-tip roast
- 1/3 cup lemon juice
- 1/3 cup soy sauce
- 1/4 cup Worcestershire sauce
- 3 tbs dried basil
- 3 tbs garlic powder
- 1.5 tbs dried parsley
- 1 tsp pepper

Directions:
1. In a blender or food processor, process soy sauce, lemon juice, Worcestershire sauce, garlic powder, basil, parsley, and pepper.
2. Rub marinade on tri-tip and refrigerate for 6 hours.
3. Roast in oven at 375 F for 1 hour.

STRACIATELLA SOUP

Ingredients:
- 6 cups fat free, low sodium chicken broth
- 2 large eggs
- 2 tbs low fat grated parmesan cheese
- 1 cup tightly pressed fresh spinach
- 1 tbs dried basil
- 1 tbs dried parsley
- salt & pepper

Directions:
1. Heat chicken broth on medium-high heat.
2. Combine and whisk together eggs, cheese, parsley, and basil.
3. Once broth begins to simmer, reduce to medium-low heat and slowly drizzle in egg mixture while stirring the broth with a fork for one minute.
4. Add spinach and season with salt and pepper to taste.

STABILIZATION PHASE RECIPES

PHILLY CHEESESTEAK

Ingredients:
- 7 oz lean roast beef, sliced into 1/2 inch strips
- 1/2 medium onion, sliced
- 1/2 green bell pepper, sliced
- 2 mushrooms, sliced
- 1 clove garlic, minced
- 1/4 cup fat free cheese (I used cheddar & mozzarella)

Directions:
1. Heat large pan on medium heat with cooking spray.
2. Saute garlic, bell peppers, onions, and mushrooms until just tender(do not overcook). Set Aside.
3. Cook roast beef on medium heat until water is rendered. Strain and set aside.
4. In the same pan, heat cooking spray over medium-high heat.
5. Re-add roast beef and vegetables. Cook until both are browned.
6. Mix in cheese and remove from heat immediately (cheese will melt fast).

DUKAN CALIFORNIA ROLLS

Ingredients:
- 3 large egg-whites, whisked
- 1/4 cup cucumber, julienned
- 1-1/2 tbs low-fat mayo
- 1/2 cup imitation crab meat, finely chopped
- 1-1/2 medium sheets of roasted seaweed
- 3 tbs low-sodium soy sauce

Directions:
1. In a small pan, heat cooking spray on medium heat.
2. Pour in egg-whites and allow it to take the round shape of the pan.
3. Cook until both sides are browned. Remove and cut egg whites into squares (1/2 inch by 1.5 inch).
4. Combine mayo with imitation crab meat and mix.
5. Cut seaweed sheets into 1.5-2 inch wide strips.
6. Place 1-2 tbs of crab meat in one section of each seaweed strip, then cucumber, & 2-3 squares of egg-whites.
7. Carefully roll the seaweed and use a toothpick to hold the roll together.
8. Serve rolls with low-sodium soy sauce.

CHICKEN CARNITAS

Ingredients:
- 6 chicken leg quarters, skin removed
- 9 garlic cloves, minced
- 1 tsp oregano
- 1 tsp chili powder
- 1/2 tsp salt
- 1/4 lime
- 1/2 tsp lemon pepper
- 1/2 tsp garlic powder
- 1/2 tsp onion powder
- 1/4 tsp pepper

Directions:
1. Preheat oven 425 F.
2. Spray a large baking dish with cooking spray.
3. Place chicken legs in dish and top with more cooking spray.
4. Combine chili powder, salt, oregano, and 2/3 of minced garlic.
5. Rub mixture on chicken and bake for 45 minutes.
6. Remove chicken from oven.
7. Use 2 forks to remove chicken meat from bone within the same baking dish and shred.
8. Mix chicken meat with juices from the baking dish.
9. Preheat medium pan on medium heat with cooking spray.
10. Add remainder of garlic and cook until fragrant.
11. Add chicken meat along with garlic powder, onion powder, lemon pepper, pepper, and 2-3 squeezes of lime juice.
12. Cook chicken until it's nice and brown and a bit crisp.

CHILI-LIME CHICKEN

Ingredients:
- 16 drumsticks, skin removed
- 1/2 cup lime juice
- 3 tbs chili powder
- 2 cloves garlic, minced
- salt & pepper
- 1 packet splenda

Directions:
1. Preheat oven 400 F.
2. Pat drumsticks dry and season with salt & pepper.
3. Place drumsticks in a large baking dish.
4. Mix remaining ingredients in a bowl and pour over chicken.
5. Cover with foil and bake for 15 minutes.
6. Remove foil and bake for another 35 minutes, basting drumsticks with juices often.
7. Remove from oven and plate drumsticks. Top with rendered sauce and garnish with lime wedges.

TIRAMISU

Ingredients:
- 1 egg yolk
- 1 egg white
- dash cream of tartar
- 10 packets splenda (and extra to sweeten layers to your liking)
- 1/4 tsp baking powder
- 1/6 cup cornstarch
- 6 tbs fat free cream cheese
- 8 tbs fat free vanilla greek yogurt
- 1/4 cup brewed espresso or any strong coffee
- 1 tbs cocoa powder
- splash of vanilla extract

Directions:
1. In a large bowl, combine and whisk together egg yolk, 10 packets splenda, 3 tbs cream cheese, 4 tbs greek yogurt, and vanilla extract.
2. Use a mixer to whisk egg white and cream of tartar until stiff.
3. Slowly add cornstarch and whisk it into the mixture.
4. Gently fold egg-white mix into egg yolk mix.
5. Pour mix into a small baking dish lined with foil.
6. Bake at 325 F for 16-20 minutes or until firm to create a sponge cake. Allow to cool.
7. Brew coffee sweetened to your liking.
8. Mix 2 tsp cocoa powder into the coffee.
9. Mix together 3 tbs cream cheese and 4 tbs greek yogurt. Sweeten mix with splenda to your liking.
10. In a souffle cup, layer coffee, sponge cake, dash of cocoa powder, and sweetened cream cheese mix (in that order).

11. Repeat these layers and finish with cream cheese mix topped with a dash of cocoa powder.
12. Refrigerate for 6 hours to allow the spongecake to soak up the coffee.

GOOD LUCK

I sincerely hope you found some of the bonus recipes utterly delicious!

If you enjoyed this book, please take a moment to share your thoughts and post a positive review on Amazon. I would greatly appreciate your support!

Good Luck in achieving your health and fitness goals, and I wish all the best to you and yours!

Benjamin Tideas

Get a FREE Kindle Book at:
http://www.plaid-enterprises.com/freebook

Visit Benjamin Tideas online:
http://www.plaid-enterprises.com/benjamin-tideas

ABOUT THE AUTHOR

Welcome! My name is Benjamin Tideas, and I write [primarily] How-To and Self-Improvement books. Growing up in middle America as a youth and a young adult, I usually made things happen in my life that required a ton of hard work (notice I didn't say smart work) but I accomplished several things I set out for including a family, higher education and a well-paying career. However, I could always feel that something was missing, and that I was an underachiever. After a somewhat devastating life event, I decided to stop and take a look at my life from ground zero - and thus began my journey into deep self-improvement. After several years in this mode, I began thinking, "You know, I just might be an acceptable source to pass on much of this new found knowledge, experience and inspiration." And so, here we are... I hope that one or more of my books may be of great help to you or someone you care about. Please feel free to let me know if I've done my job. =)

www.ingramcontent.com/pod-product-compliance
Lightning Source LLC
Chambersburg PA
CBHW070506290526
45790CB00003B/1117